FIGHT MY JOURNEY

WRITTEN BY
J'IOR PRINCETON

ILLUSTRATED BY
ASHLEY MAE PANCHO

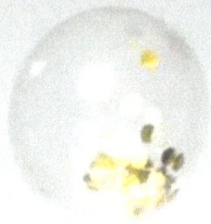

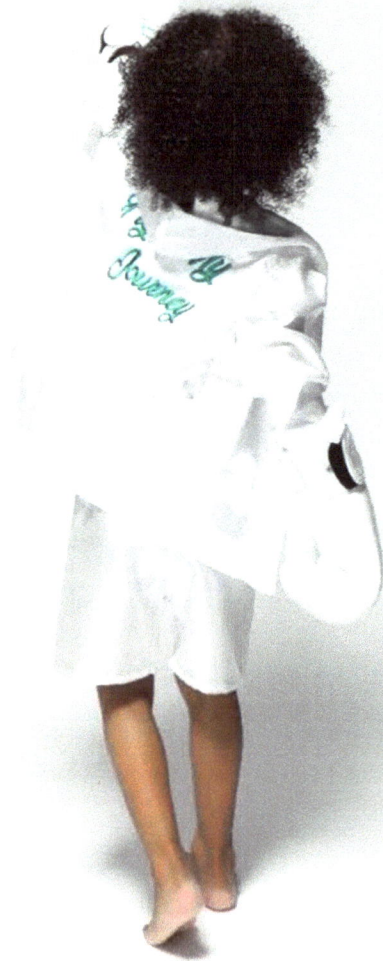

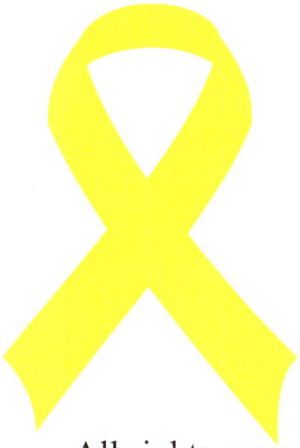

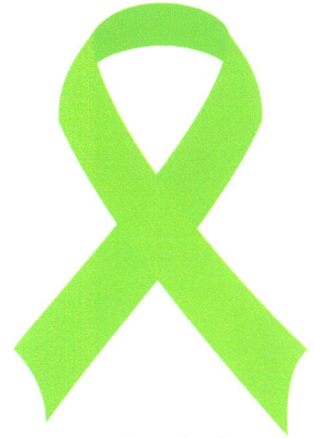

Copyright © 2021 J'ior Princeton

Printed in the United States of America

EDITOR: Stacey M. Robinson (Kya Publishing Canada)

COVER DESIGN: Chamika Dinesh

ILLUSTRATOR: Ashley Mae Pancho

PAGE DESIGN: Osamudiamenabdul

CONTRIBUTIONS: ElevatedWaves Publishing Corp.

PUBLISHER: Fight My Journey LLC

ISBN: 978-0-578-97309-8

Library of Congress Control Number: 2021917028

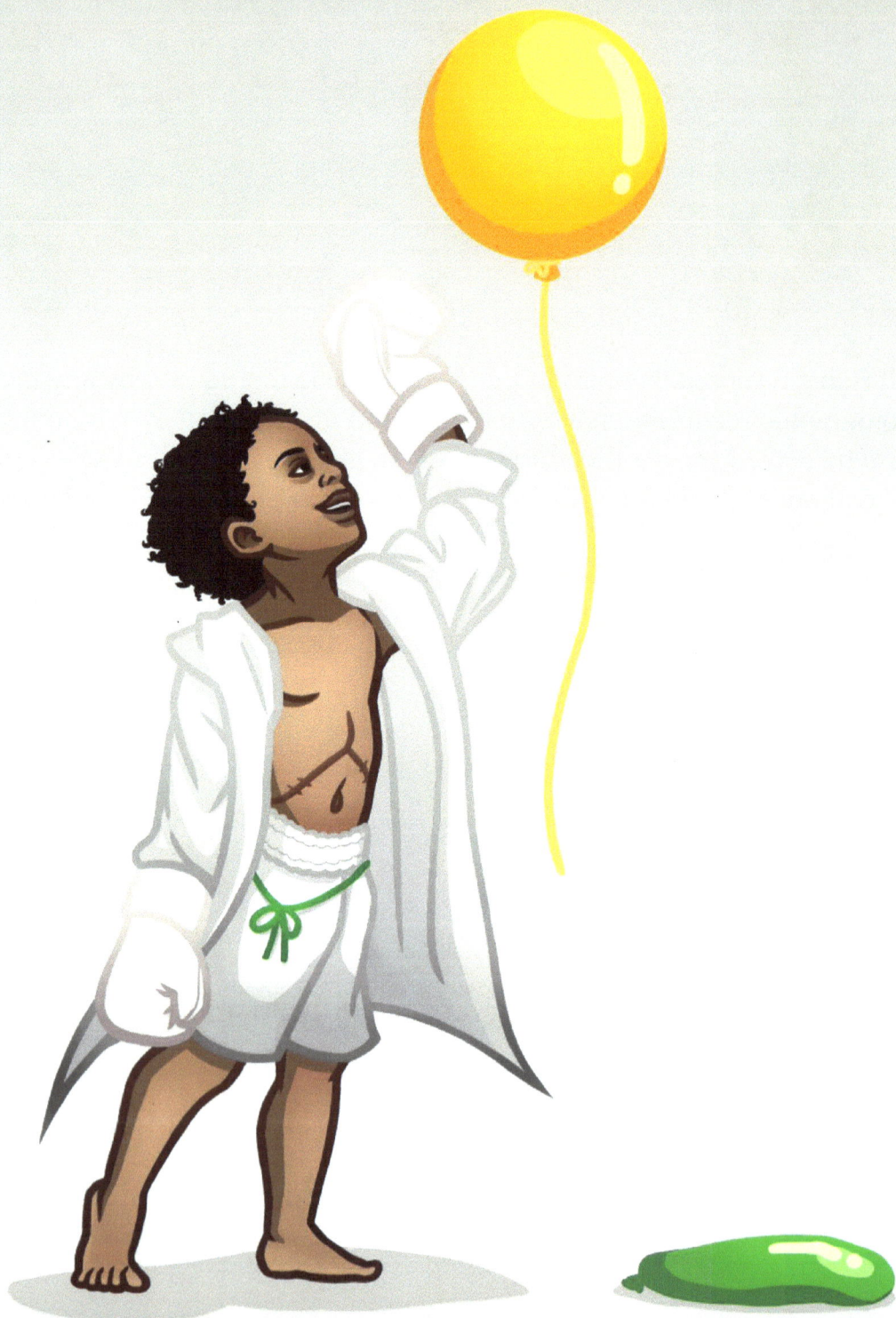

Hello friends! My Name is J'ior.

My mom loves to tell people a great story about how I became a warrior, and how I was given a second chance at life.

I thought it would be a great idea to share my story with the world, to teach my friends, and to let you know how strong you can be too!

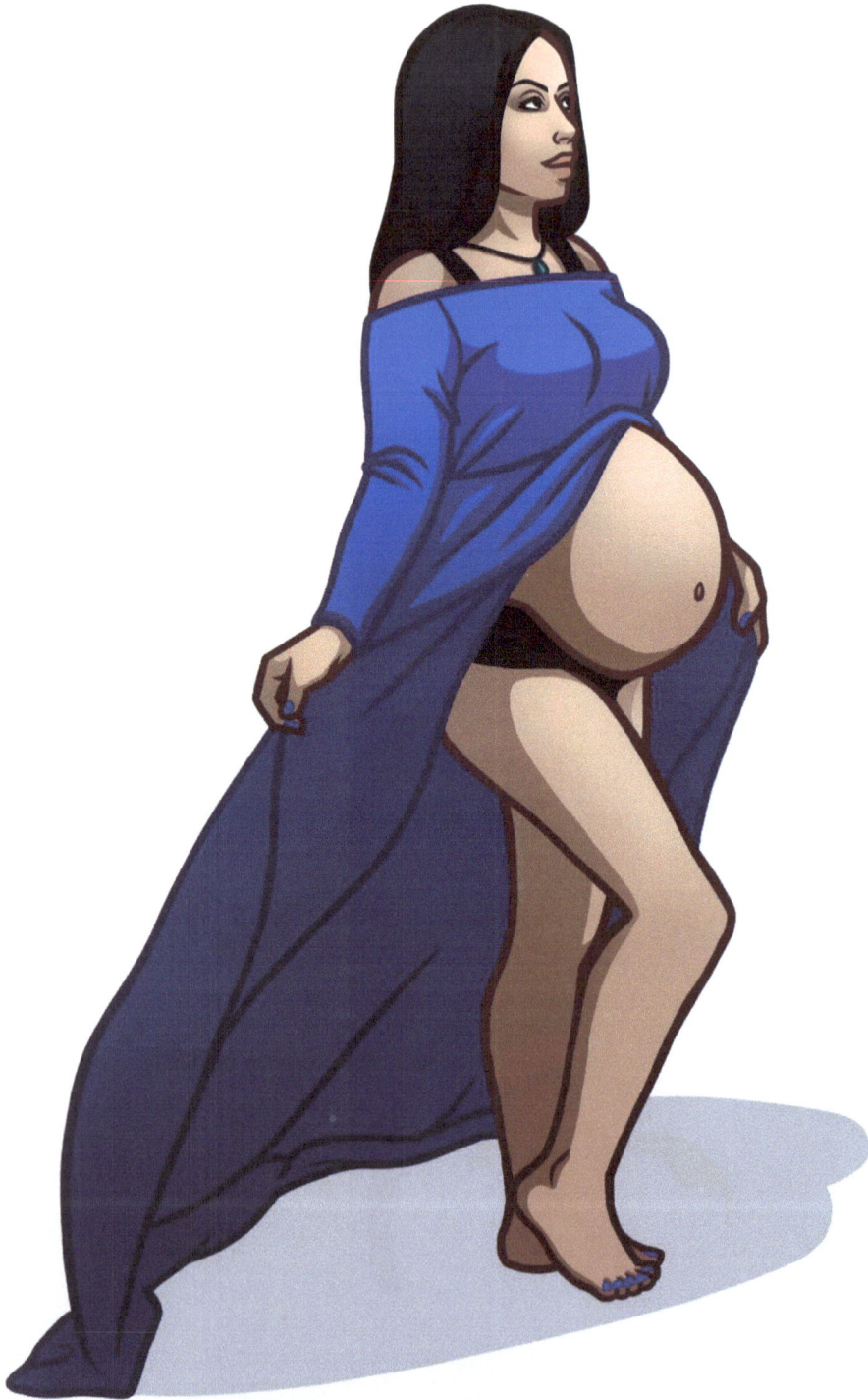

I was born on New Year's Eve in the year 2017. My mom said it was a coooold snowy day. There was so much snow outside that Mommy said she could barely see — the snow covered the trees and the cars!

It was so bad that Mommy had to call an ambulance to drive us to the hospital, because I was ready for the world!

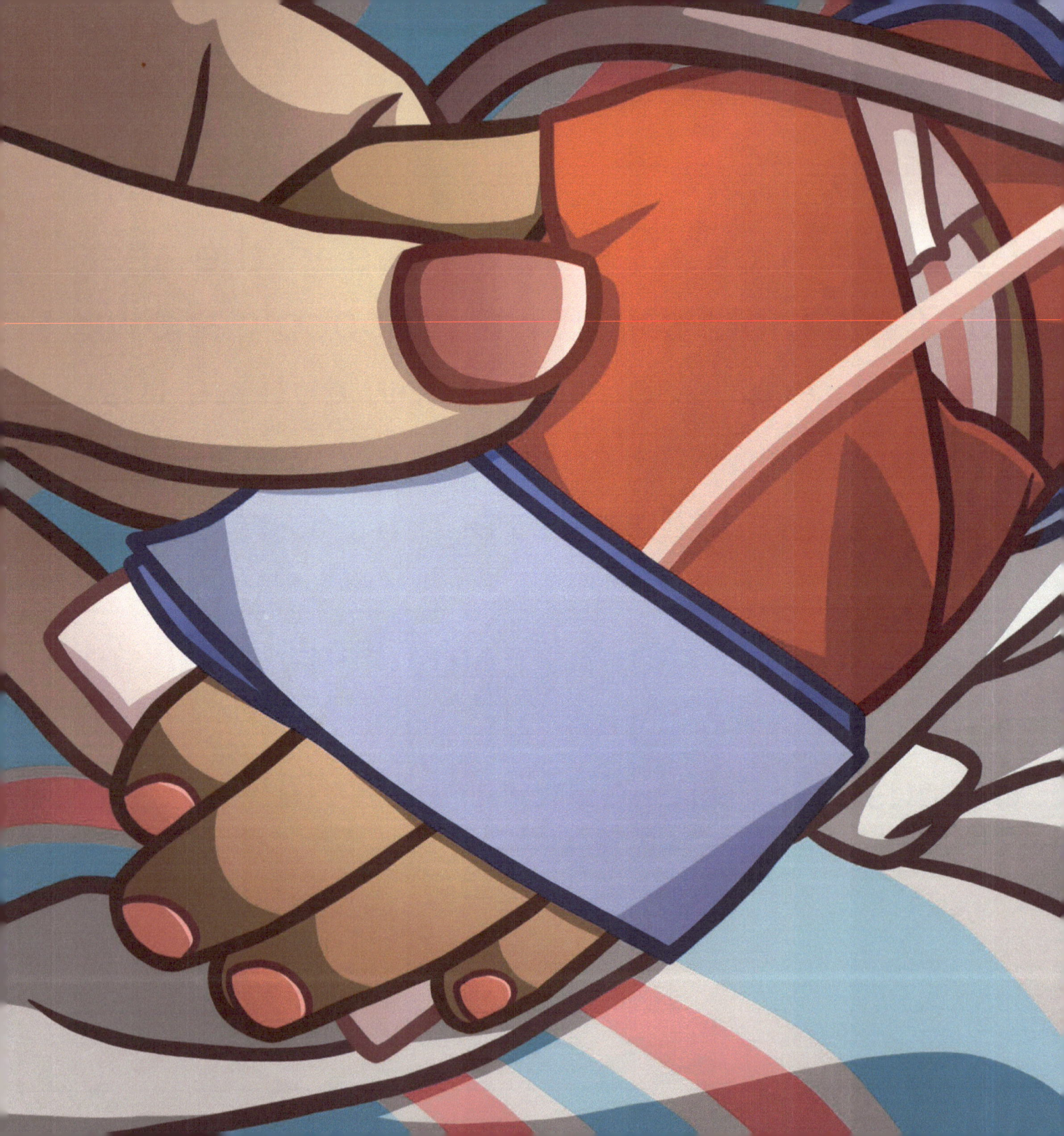

After I was born, even though the doctor said I was discharged and I could go home from the hospital, my mom felt there was something wrong with me... so instead of taking me home, she took me to another hospital.

I was only 2 days old, and I had to go to a different hospital for more testing... to make sure everything was OK.

The hospital was big with a nice indoor play area. Even though I was just a newborn baby, Mommy still took me down to the playroom for story time and music every single day.

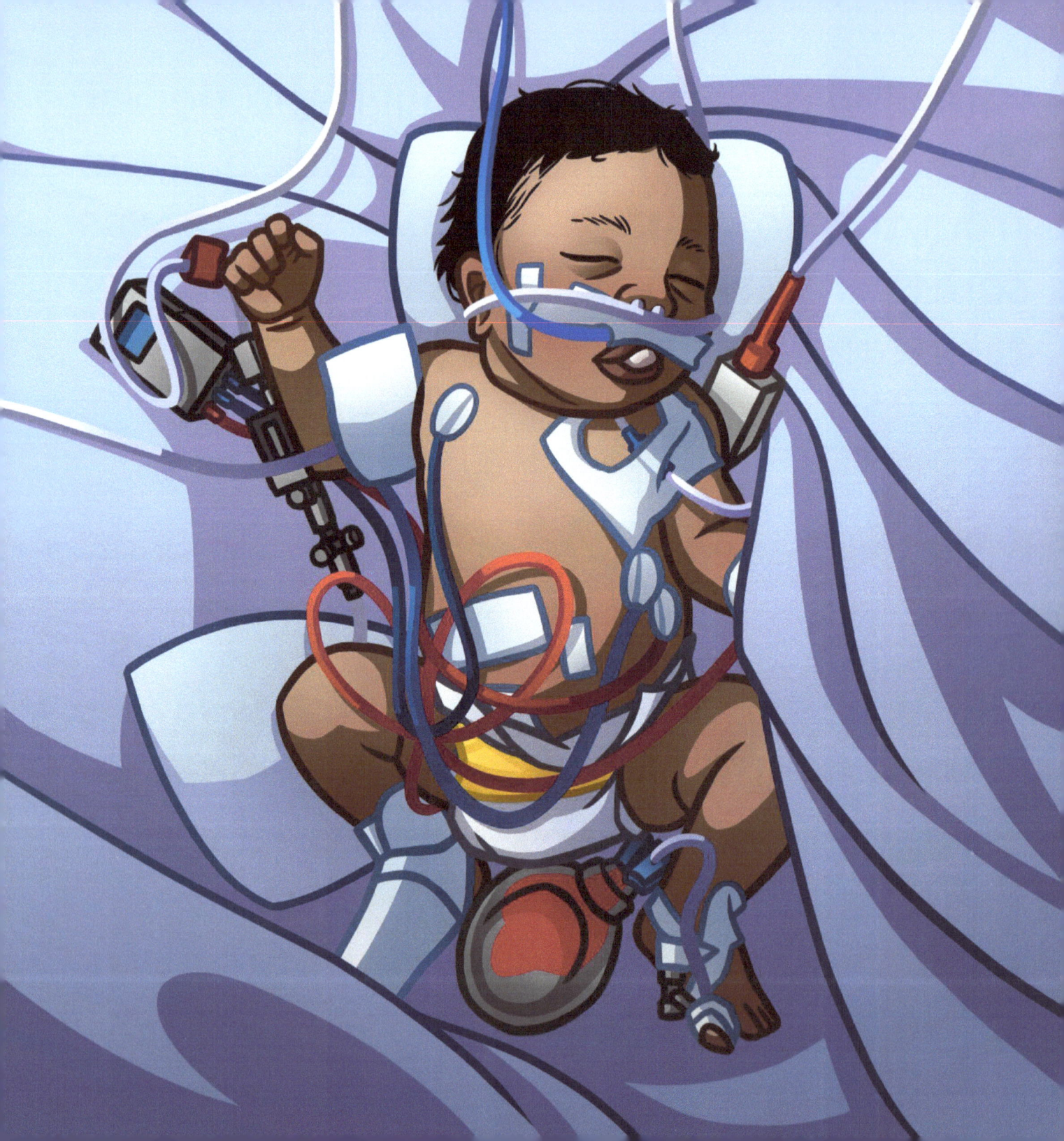

By day 23, after all their testing, the doctors learned that I had a liver disease called Biliary Atresia and that I had to have an emergency surgery called a Kasia.

The Kasia surgery is a 5-to-7-hour long procedure that was not going to cure me from liver damage... but it was going to delay me from having a liver transplant right away.

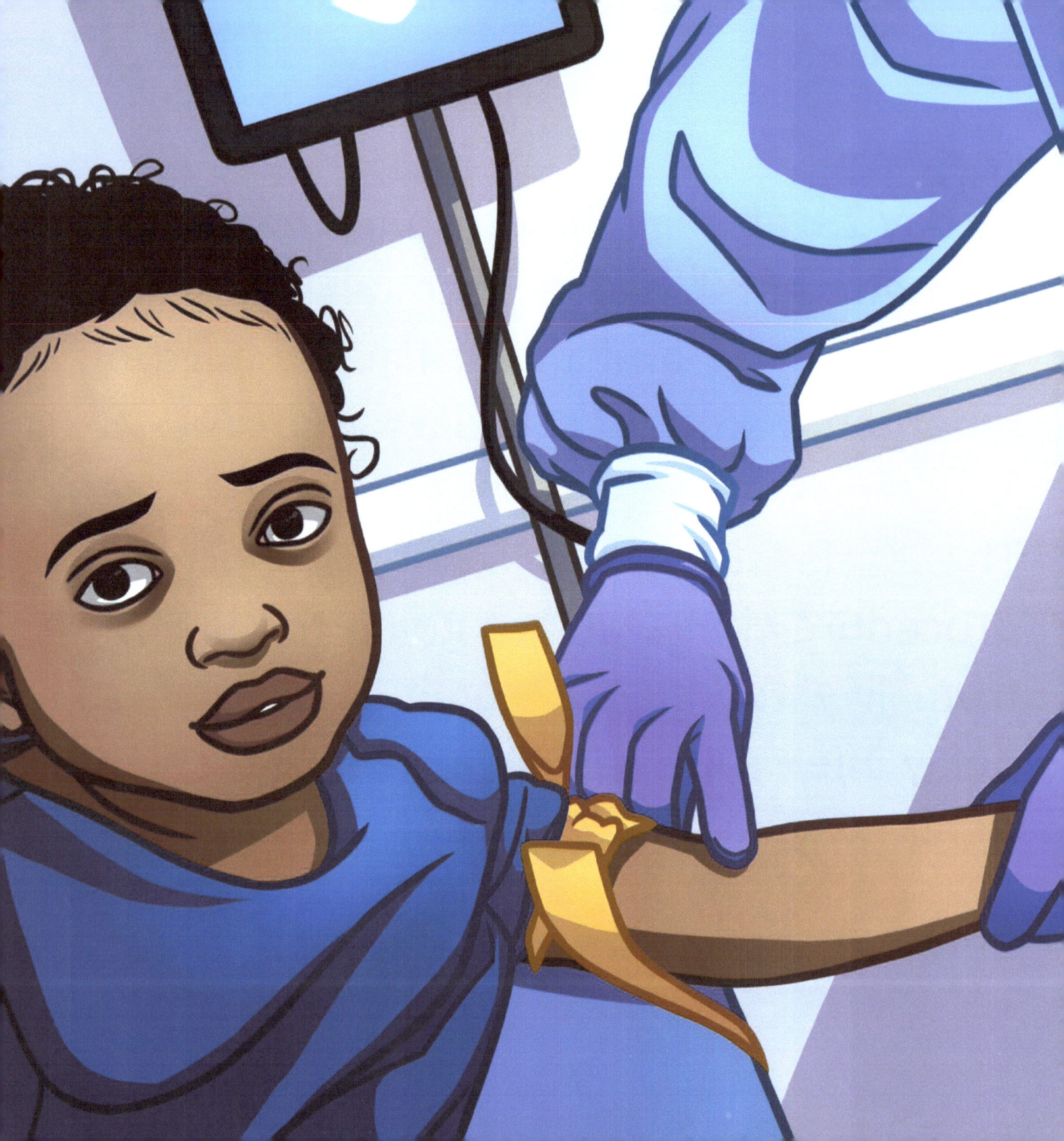

After months and months going in and out... and in and out... and back in and out again of the hospital, I was told that the my Kasia procedure was not working!

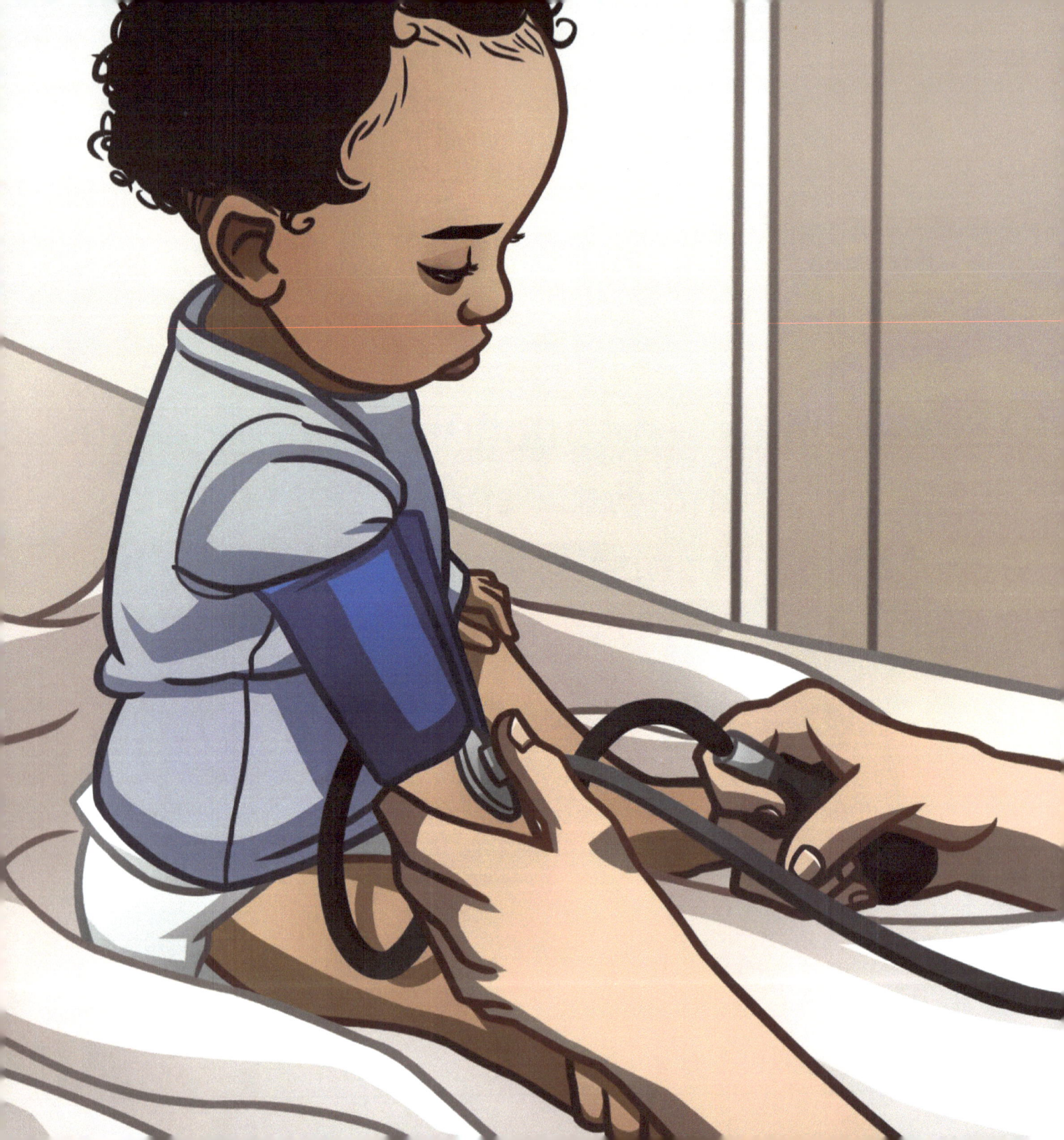

They said I had to be placed on a list to wait for another procedure: a transplant.

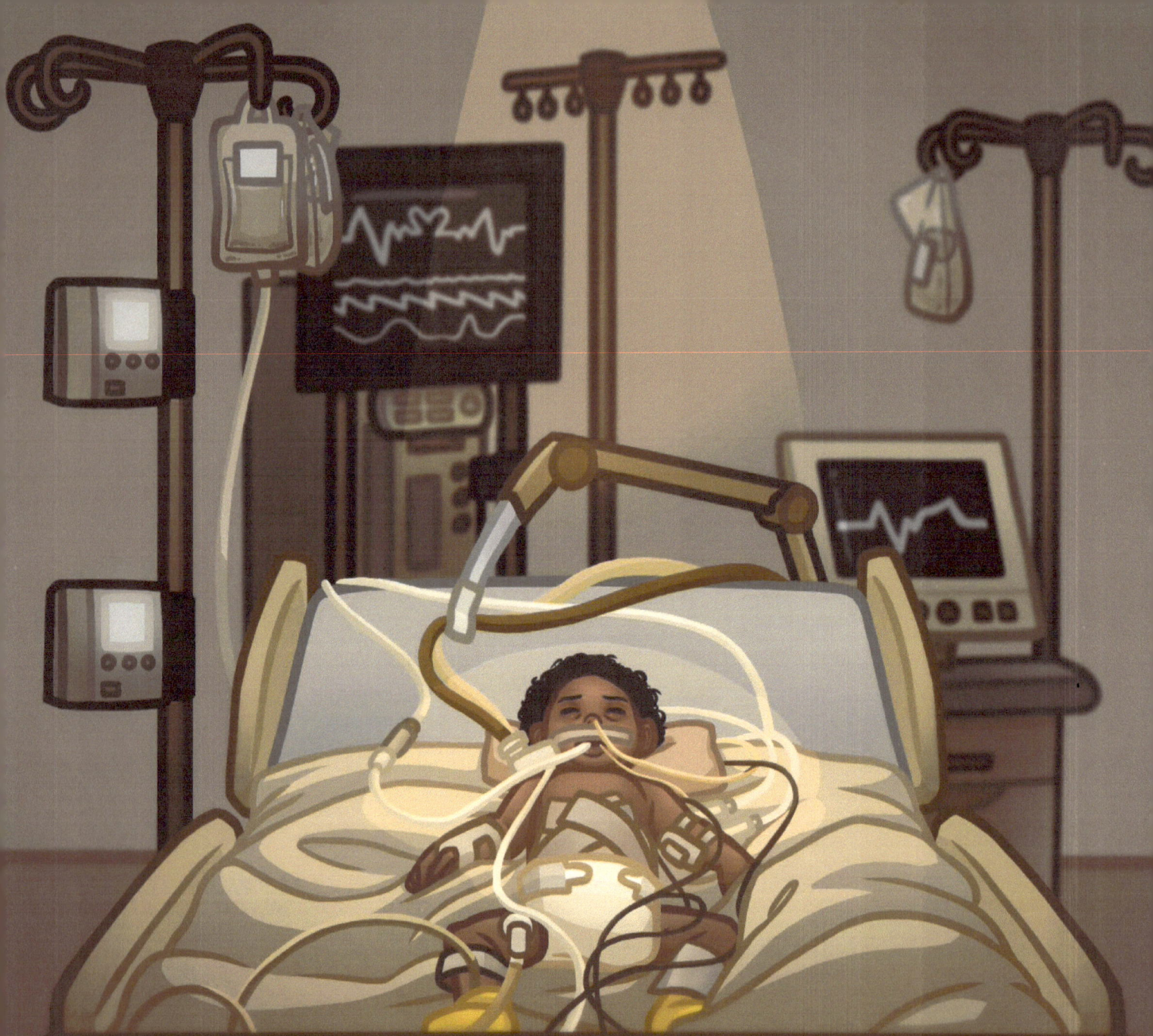
Liver Transplant 6/6/19

Finally... when I was 17 months old, my name was next on the list! It was my turn to receive a liver transplant and get my second chance at life!

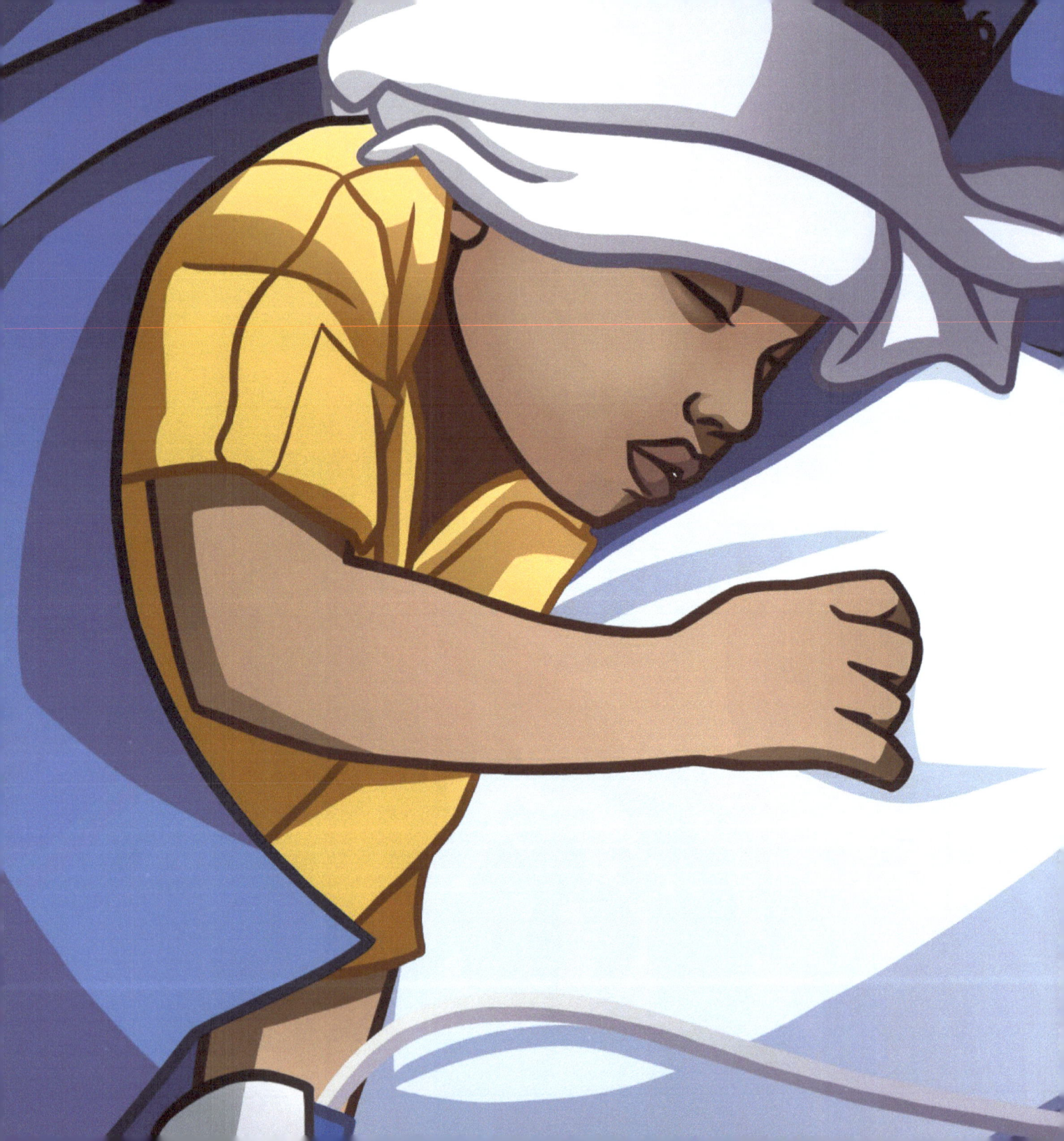

After the transplant, things weren't fixed right away. My mom wanted to take me home to celebrate...but I now had another disease called C-M-V.

Because of the new CMV disease, I had to stay in the hospital (AGAIN) for many, many more months to get treatment.

CMV stands for Cytomegalovirus. Let's try to say this word together... it's a big one: cy-to-me-ga-lo-vi-rus.

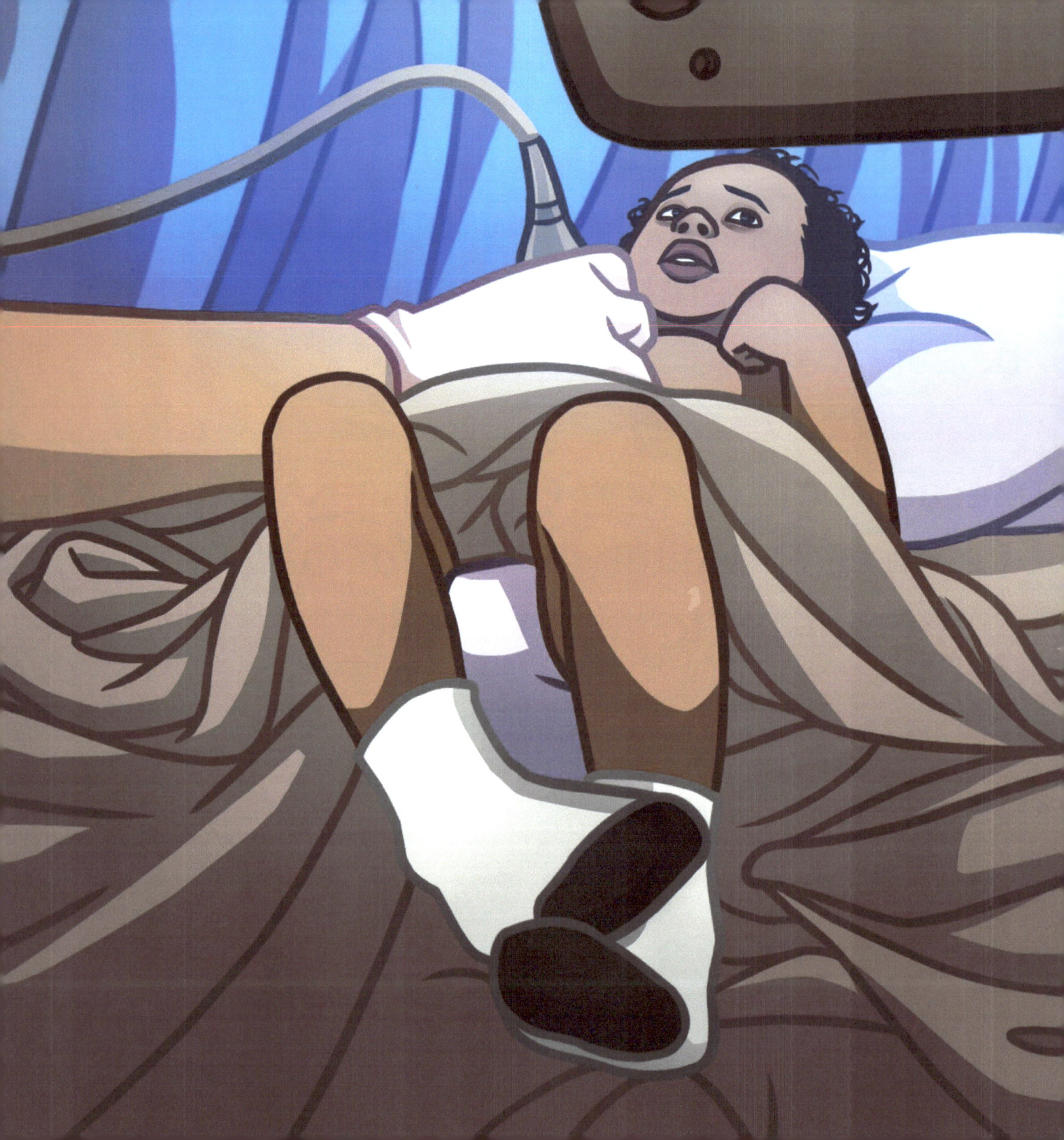

What is CMV? My mom said it is a virus found everywhere around the world. CMV is almost like some other viruses... like the chickenpox (have you ever had that itchy situation?) and another virus called infectious mononucleosis... that's another big word, so let's just call it "mono" for short.

The doctor said that once someone has CMV in their body, it stays there for life. Most people with CMV don't even get sick, and they don't even know that they've been infected!

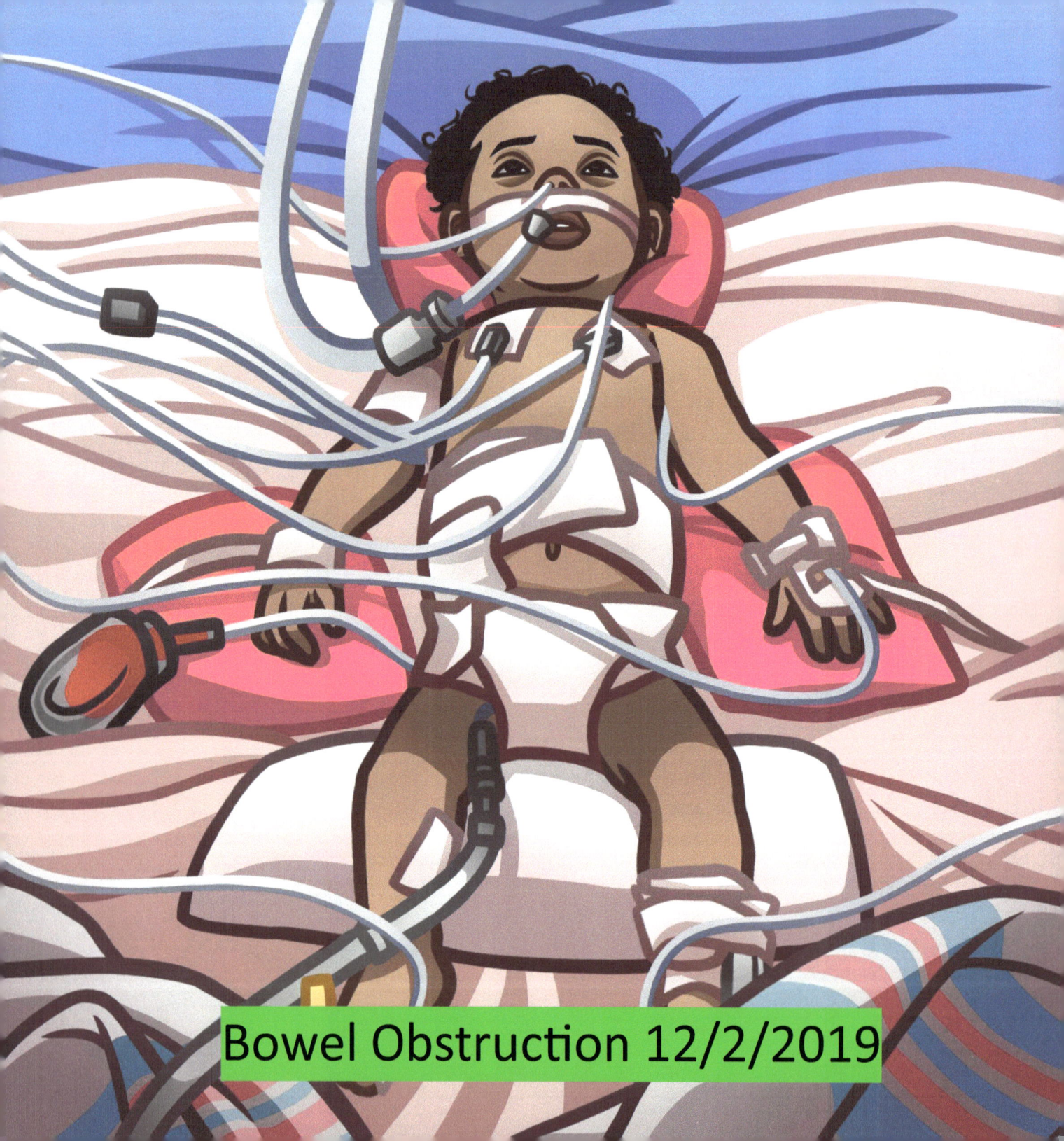

Bowel Obstruction 12/2/2019

The reason I got sick is because I was very, very young. Since I was infected with the virus when I was a baby, it was very serious.

The virus can be bad for babies and also bad for people with weak immune systems. If you have a weak immune system, it means that it is easier to get sick because your body is not able to fight against bacteria, viruses, or other things that might cause infections.

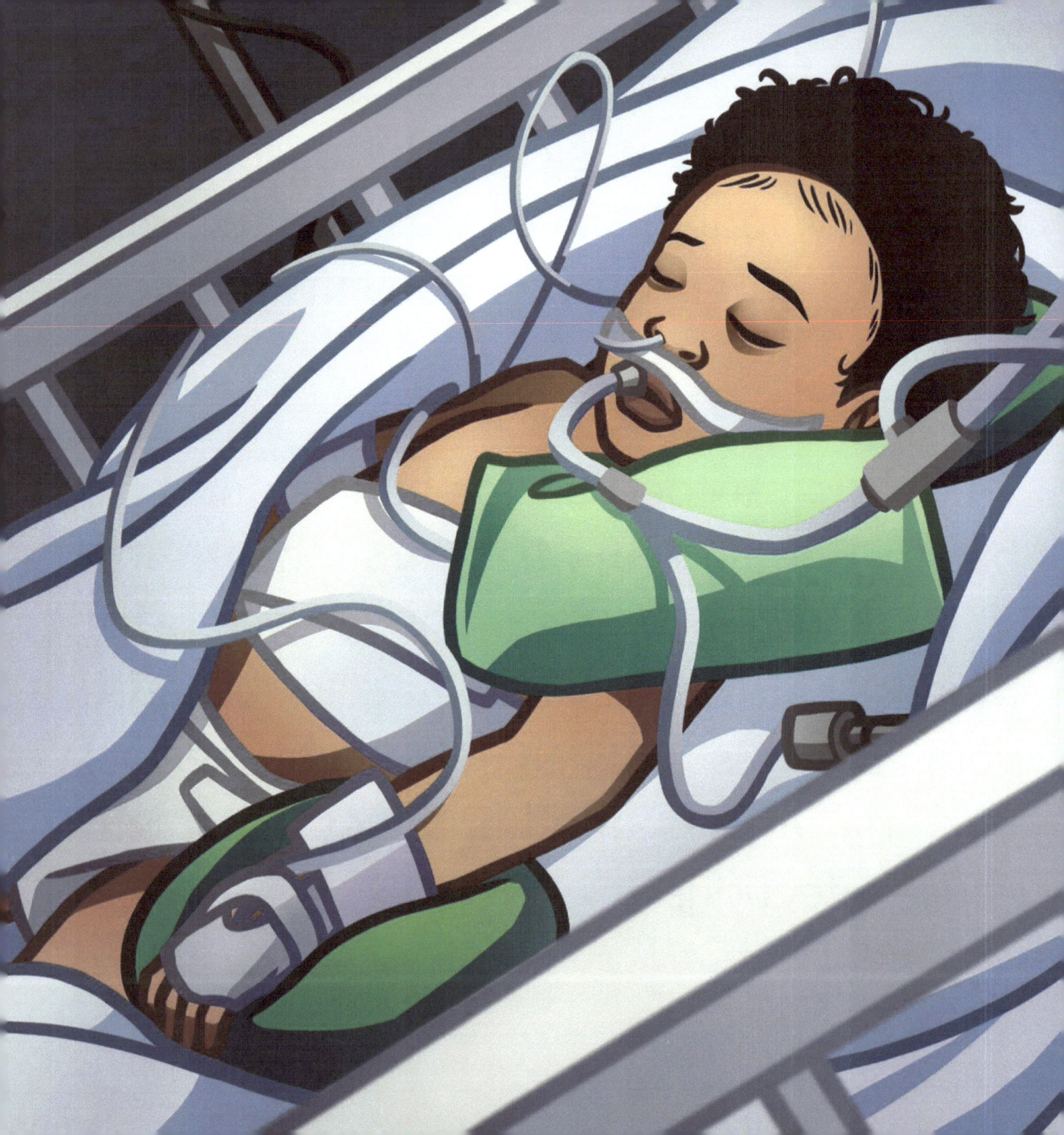

My mom was excited when the CMV cleared up when I was 21 months old: what a relief! I was able to go home... I was discharged (AGAIN) from the hospital!

I was only out of the hospital for 2 months... before I went back (AGAIN) because I had something they called severe Bowel Obstruction.

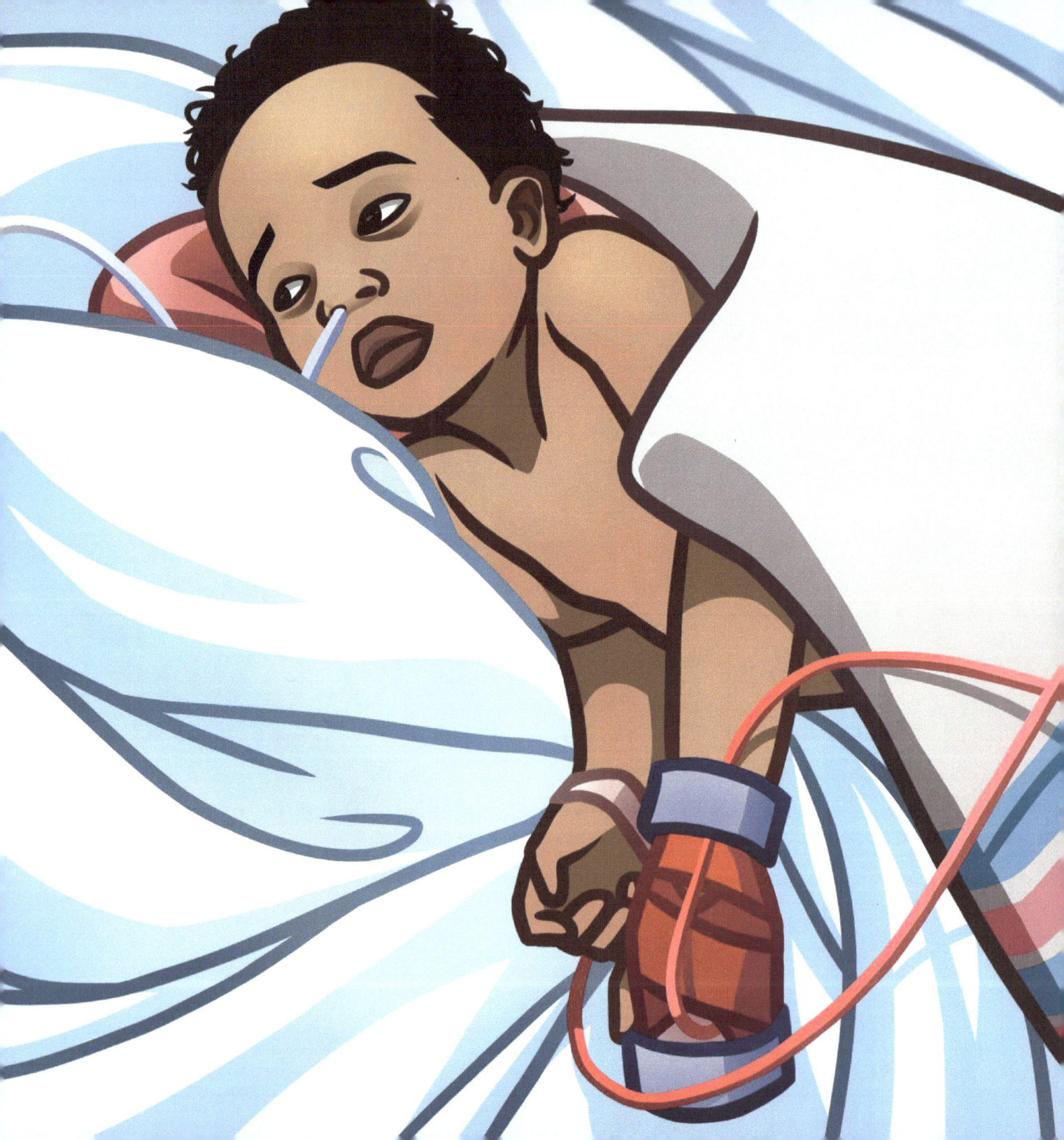

This was frustrating, but my mom stayed strong! My family stayed strong! Everyone believed that things would soon be OK, and that I would return home... AGAIN!

My Auntie Eva (Mommy's big sister), my Auntie Stephani (Mommy's childhood friend), my big cousin Boobie, (Mommy's cousin), my Godmother Marvalyn, and our Pastor Reverend Thomas were my mom's biggest support system.

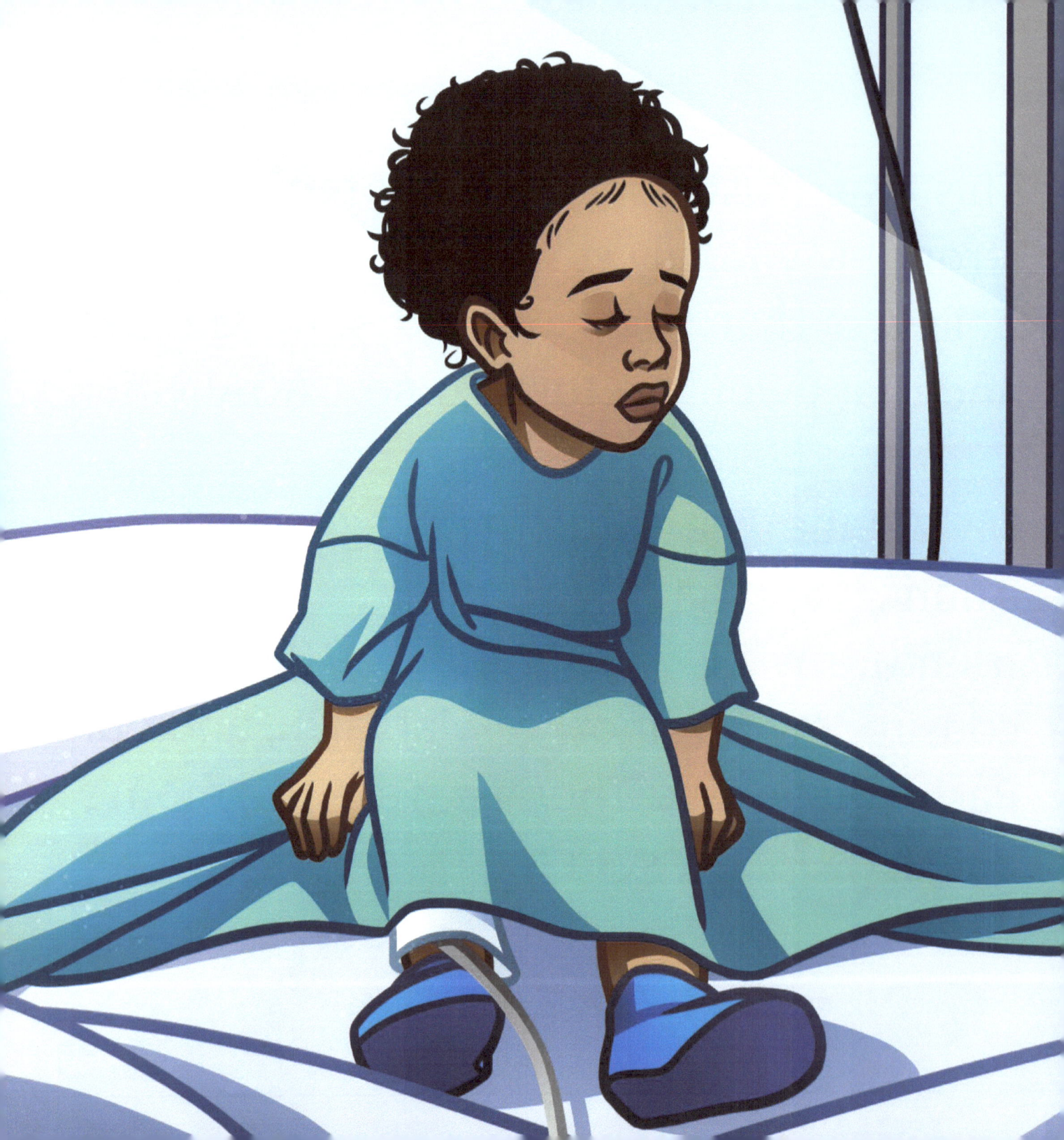

So, I was back in the hospital at 23 months old, and another disease came around... this time it wasn't in my body, but it was spreading around the world. This was called COVID-19.

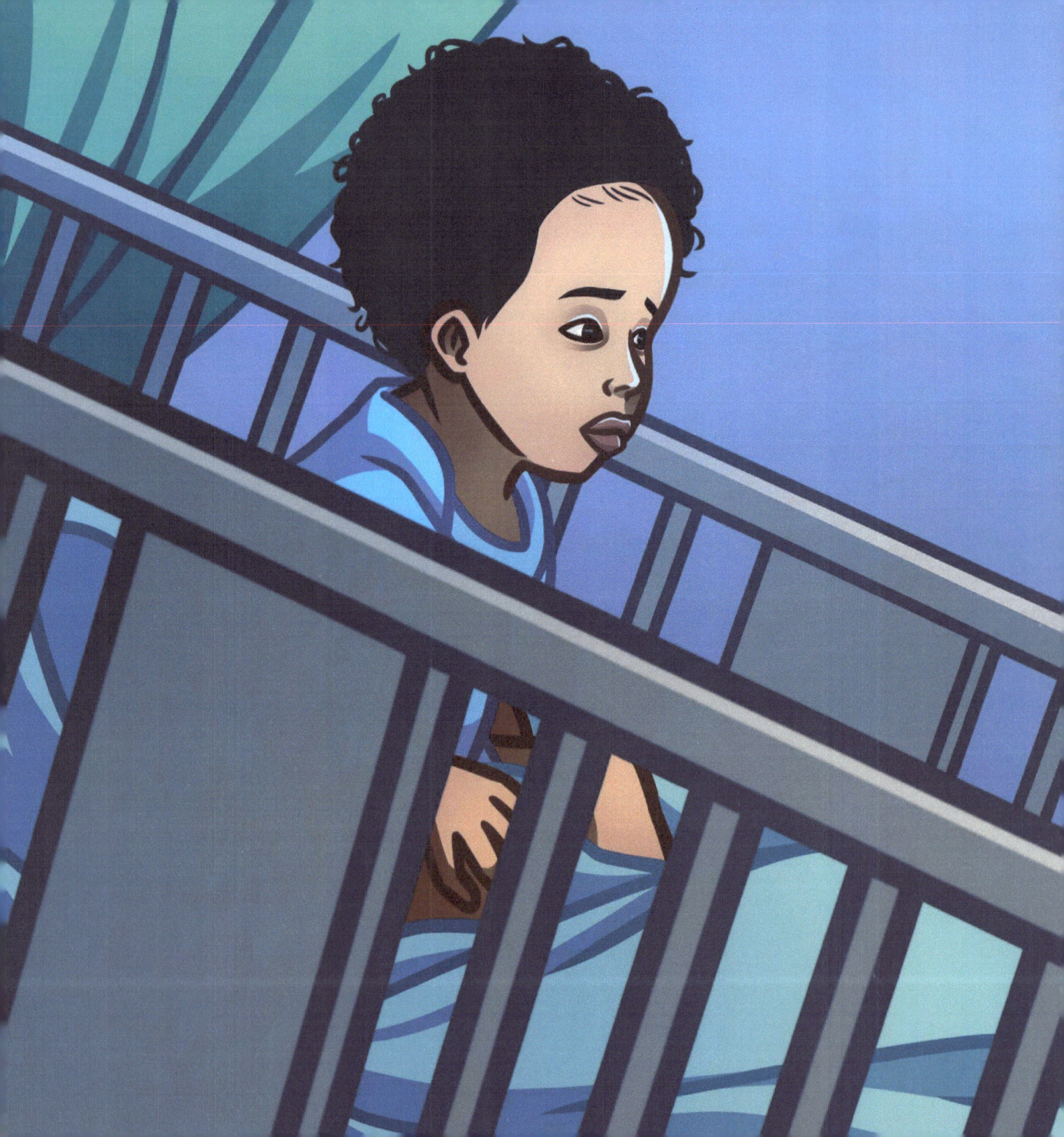

When COVID-19 started to spread, everything became more difficult... everywhere... for everyone!

Because my immune system was compromised, Mommy had to quit her job during the COVID-19 crisis. She worked in a facility that was infested with COVID-19 and if she stayed there, it would have put me at risk.

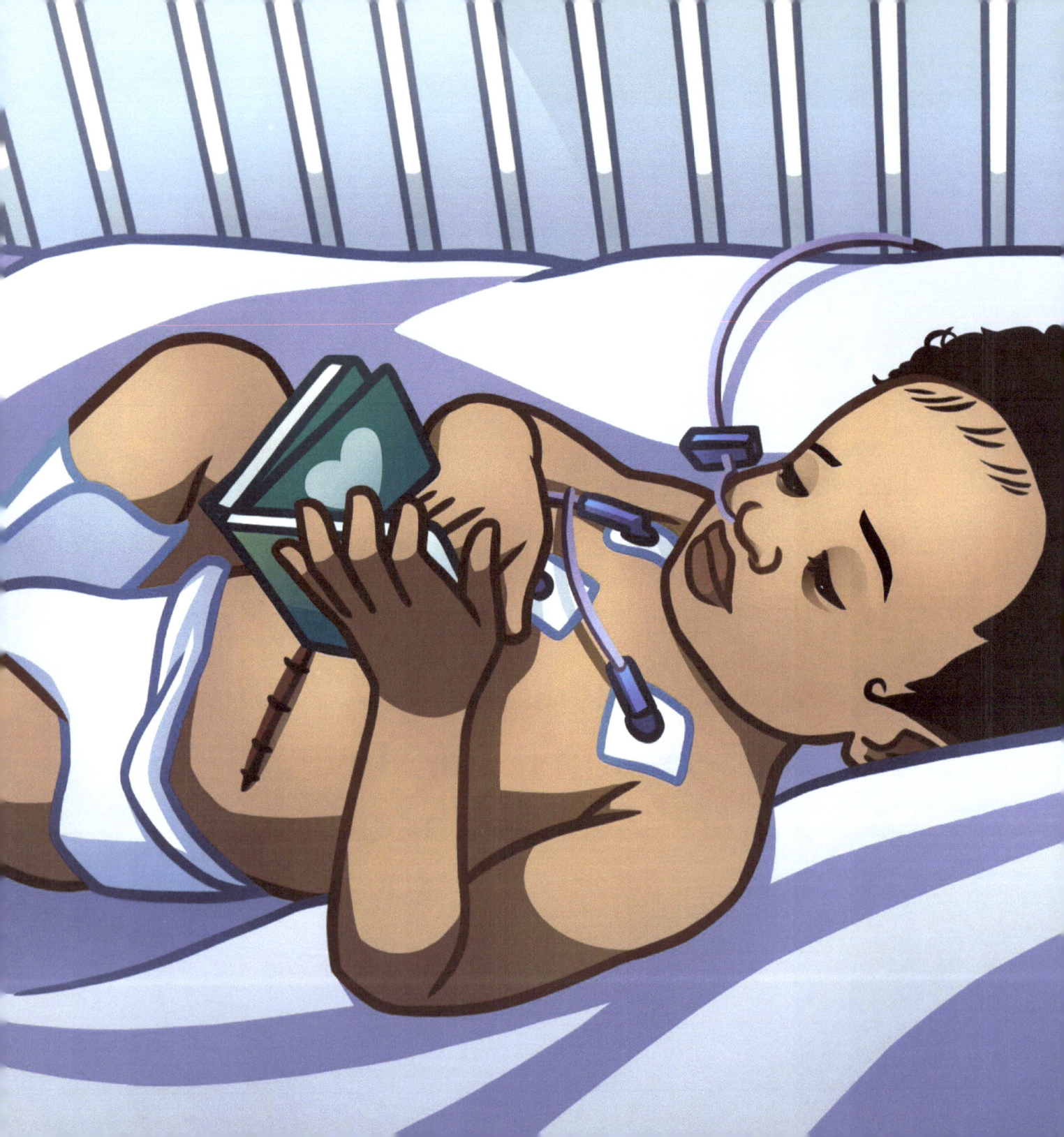

I was not able to go to daycare, because of COVID-19.

I was not able to be out in large groups because of COVID-19.

Because I had some health challenges, I was what they call "high risk" and had to be very careful about who and what I was around.

My mom had to keep me safe, and make sure I was not exposed to anything... especially to COVID-19!

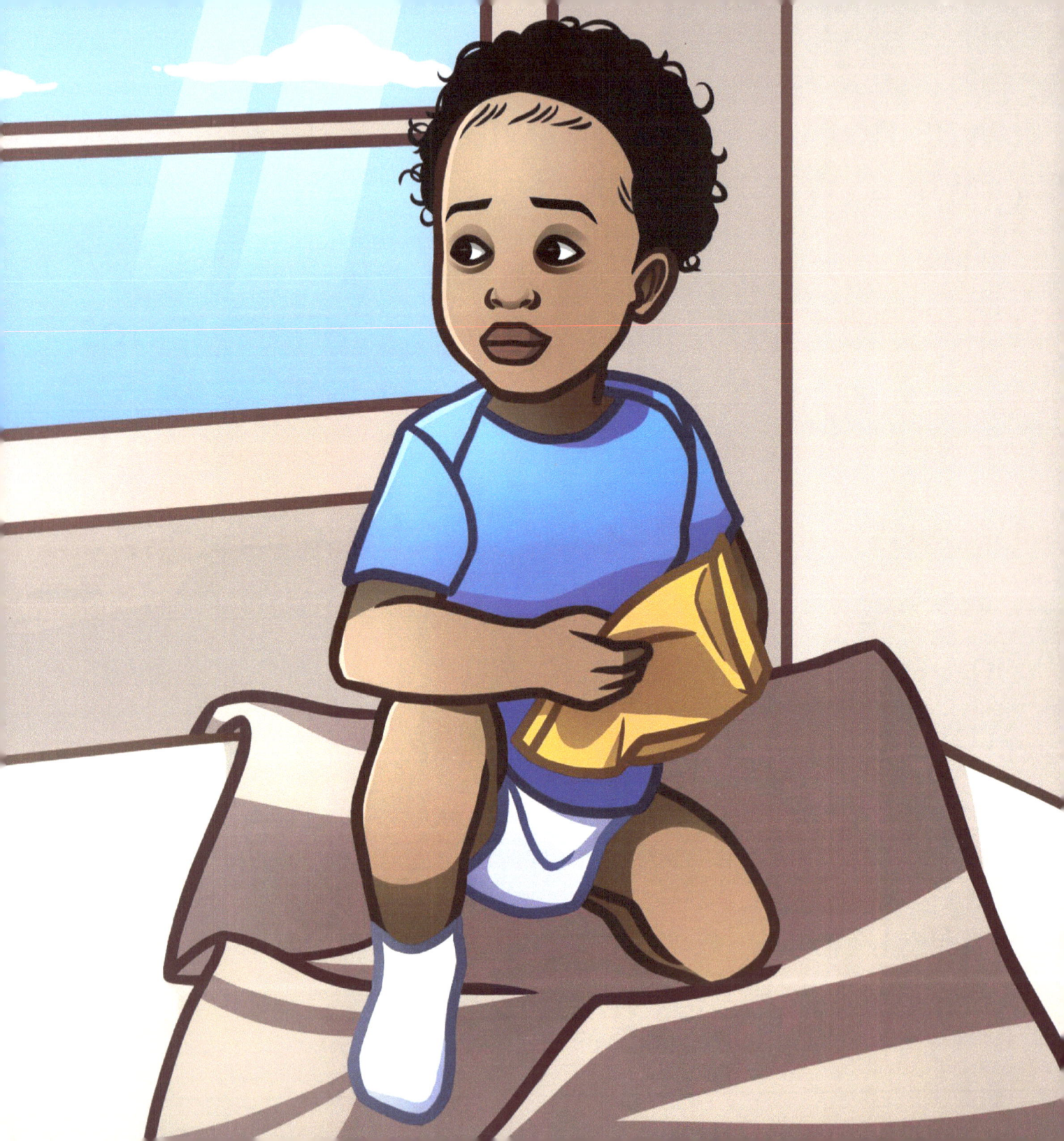

Even before the ==pandemic==, I was isolated from others to stay healthy and safe! After COVID-19... it was even more important for me to stay protected from illness.

To keep me safe, Mommy had to have my family come sit with me so she could shop, run errands, and do small jobs to help with bills (because she was unable to work full time).

Mommy never let me go anywhere, and the people who sat with me often got COVID-19 testing done because they were also high risk and in quarantine.

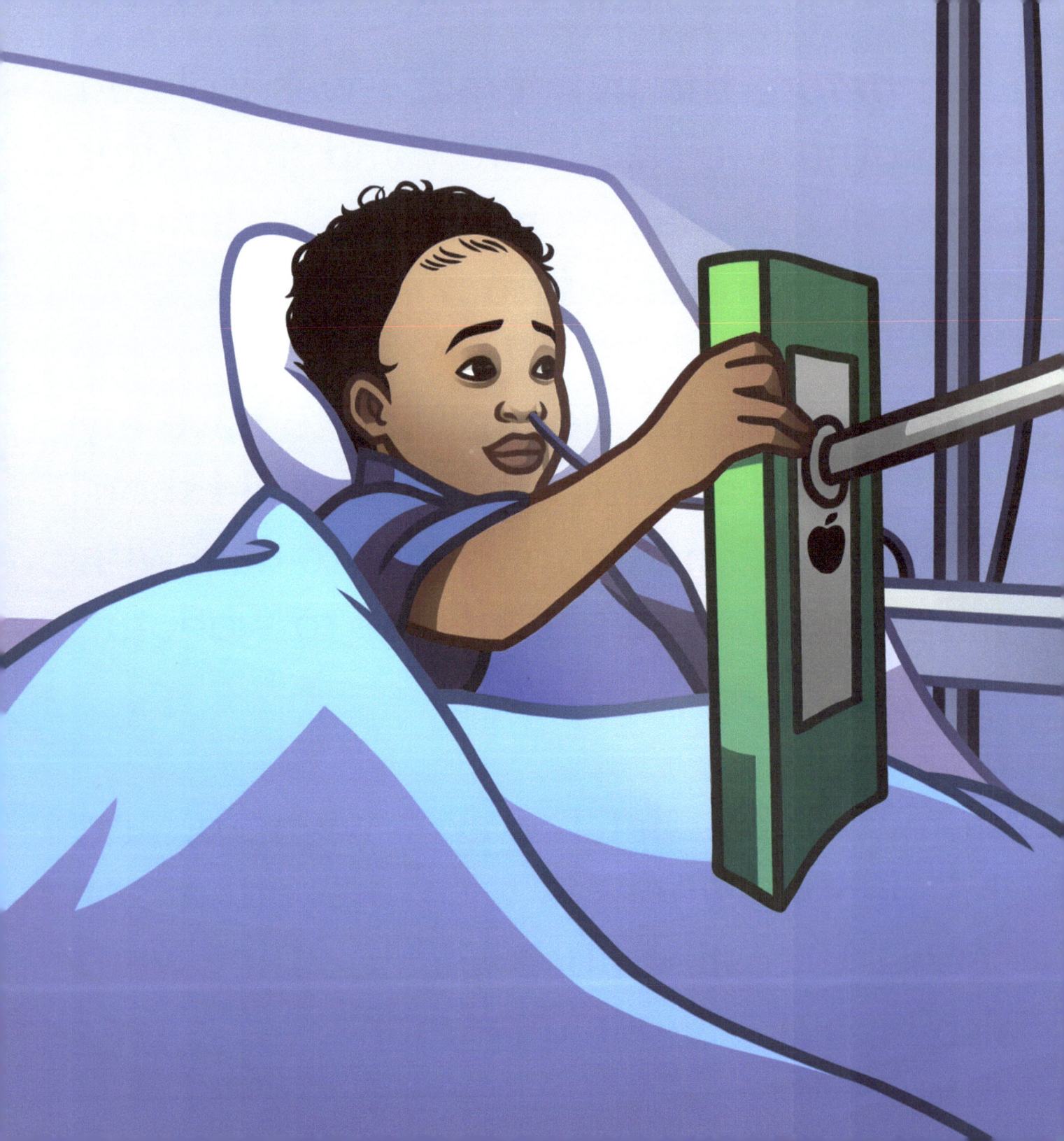

Now I am almost 4 years old (44 months), and I am doing well!

I can travel and go to half-day pre-school... as long as I wear my mask the whole time. Did you ever have to wear a mask?

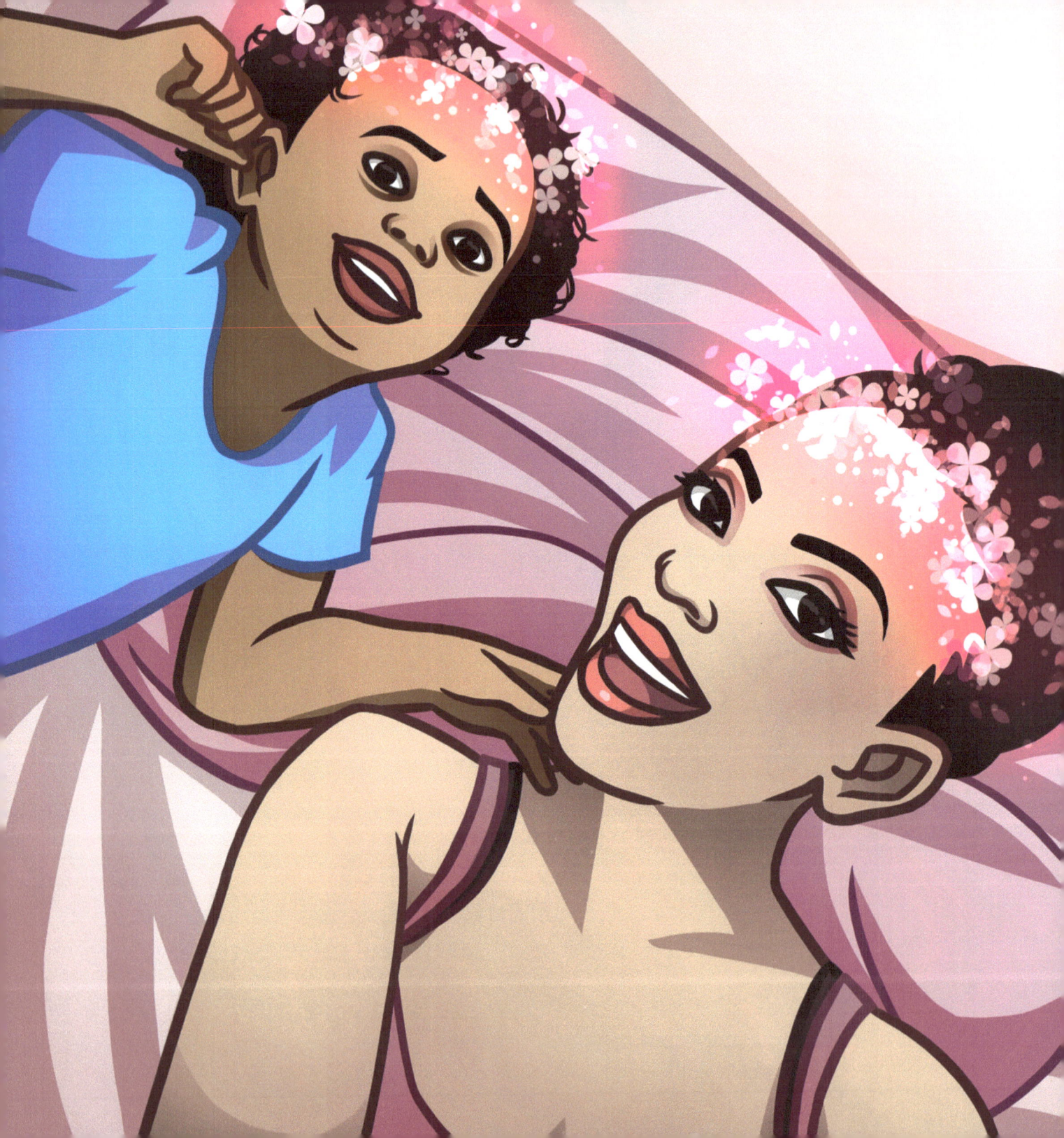

My mother says I am a true warrior! The doctors say I am a true warrior! I know that I am a true warrior, and I am no longer fighting...thanks to my donor!

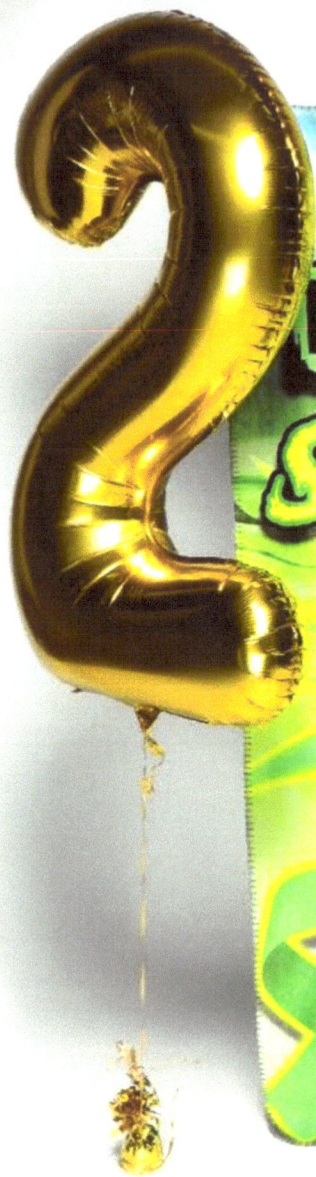

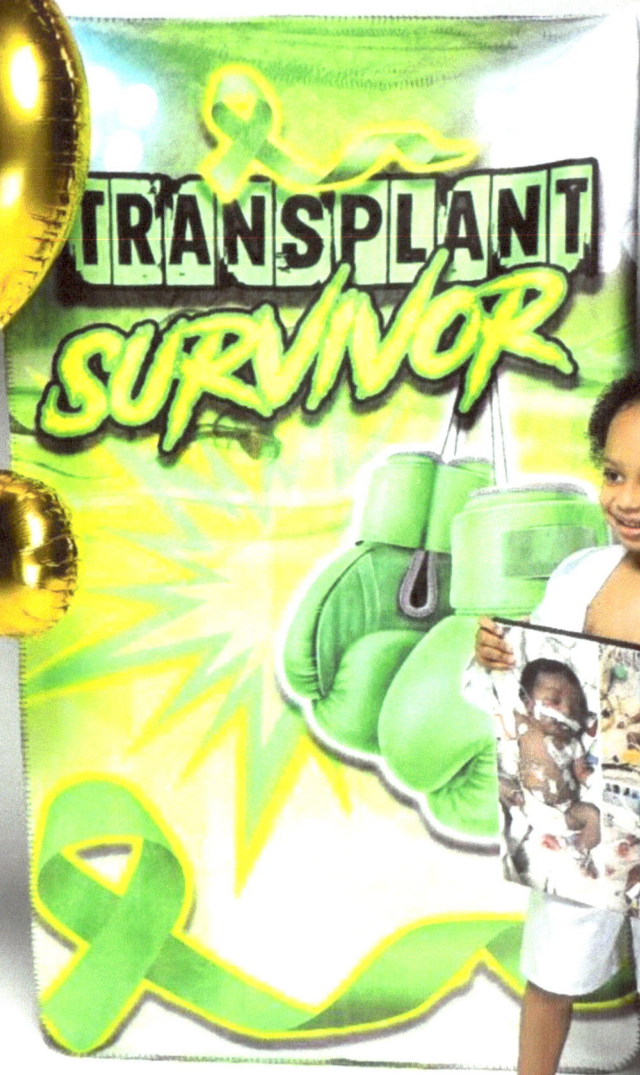

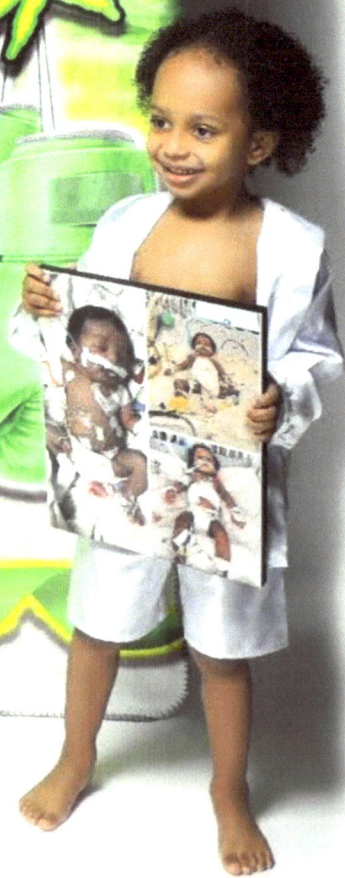

My story, and other illnesses and diseases like COVID-19 teach us how to stay safe. So when you hear about hospitals, and medication, and procedures, and surgeries with your family, your friends, your teachers, your neighbors, or other people you love... remember they will push through, and we can all be warriors together!

I would like you to remember that just because someone gets sick doesn't mean their life is over! We should always be loved, respected, and treated like human beings...when we're sick, and when we're healthy!

We all just need a little more love!

Biliary Atresia

A condition in infants where the bile ducts (outside and inside the liver) are scarred and blocked. Bile can't flow into the intestine, so it builds up in the liver and damages it. The damage leads to scarring, and a loss of liver tissue and function.

Bowel Obstruction

When either your small or large intestine is partly or completely blocked. The blockage prevents food, fluids, and gas from moving through the intestines in the normal way.

Chicken Pox

An infectious disease causing a mild fever and an itchy, red rash that breaks out on the face, scalp, chest, back and (sometimes) on the arms and legs.

COVID-19

An infectious disease that can trigger a respiratory tract infection. It can affect your upper respiratory tract (sinuses, nose, and throat) or lower respiratory tract (windpipe and lungs). It spreads the same way other viruses do—mainly through person-to-person contact.

Cytomegalovirus (CMV)

A kind of herpes virus which usually produces very mild symptoms (such as fever or fatigue) in an infected person. It may cause severe nerve damage in people with weakened immune systems and in the newborn (such as pneumonia, hepatitis, retinitis, brain inflammation, or seizures).

Discharged

To allow (someone) to leave a hospital.

Disease

A particular abnormal condition that negatively affects the structure or function of all or part of a person.

Donor
A person who provides blood for transfusion, or an organ or tissue for transplantation.

Exposed
To cause someone to be vulnerable or at risk.

High-Risk
Being particularly subject to potential danger or hazard.

Immune System
A complex network of cells, tissues, organs, and the substances they make that helps the body fight infections and other diseases.

Infectious Mononucleosis (Mono)

Often called the "kissing disease," the virus is spread through saliva. You can get it through kissing, but you can also be exposed by sharing a glass or food utensils with someone who has mono.

Kasia

The liver has ducts so that the bile it produces can drain into the intestine and help with the digestion of food. If these ducts are blocked, the Kasai procedure is a way to surgically bypass them and prevent liver damage. It is often the preferred treatment for biliary atresia.

Liver Transplant

A surgical procedure that removes a liver that no longer functions properly (liver failure) and replaces it with a healthy liver from a deceased donor or a portion of a healthy liver from a living donor.

Medication

A drug used to diagnose, cure, treat, or prevent disease.

Pandemic

An epidemic of an infectious disease that has spread across a large region—for instance, multiple continents or worldwide—affecting a substantial number of people.

Procedure

An activity directed at (or performed on) an individual with the object of improving health, treating disease or injury, or making a diagnosis.

Quarantining/Quarantine

A strict isolation imposed to prevent the spread of disease.

Testing

A medical procedure performed to detect, diagnose, or monitor diseases, disease processes, susceptibility, or to determine a course of treatment.

Treatment

Medical care given to a patient for an illness or injury.

Warrior

A brave or experienced soldier or fighter... like J'ior!

FIGHT MY JOURNEY

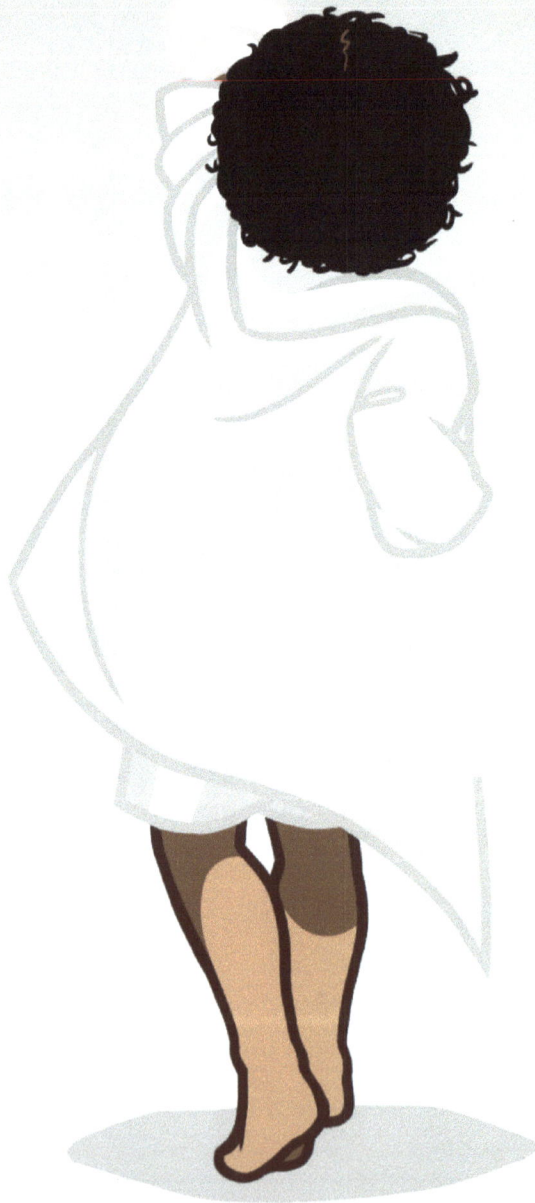

FOLLOW MY JOURNEY ON

INSTAGRAM: @FightMyJourney

FACEBOOK: FightMy Journey

USE YOUR
SMARTPHONE
CAMERA TO SCAN
MY CODES: SCAN,
TAP AND FOLLOW

TIKTOK:

www.ingramcontent.com/pod-product-compliance
Lightning Source LLC
Chambersburg PA
CBHW060817270326
41930CB00002B/74